Bodybuilding For Women

A Step-By-Step Bodybuilding Guide For Women Training Guide To Become Stronger And Fitter Than Ever

Table of Contents

Want more books?

Would you love books delivered straight to your inbox every week?

Free?

How about non-fiction books on all kinds of subjects?

We send out e-books to our loyal subscribers every week to download and enjoy!

All you have to do is join! It's so easy!

Just visit the link at the end of this book to sign up and then wait for your books to arrive!

Introduction

I want to thank you and congratulate you for purchasing the book, "Bodybuilding For Women: *A Step-By-Step Bodybuilding Guide For Women Training Guide To Become Stronger And Fitter Than Ever"*

Everyone knows how important it is to be healthy and fit in order to live a good life. But there are too many people who do nothing to get this. Now that you have downloaded this book, you are definitely heading in the right direction.

A healthy body will help you live a healthier and happier life. You can only get that kind of body if you are willing to work for it. And although it may seem hard to follow the steps, the result is definitely worth it.

You just need to be determined and you will soon see your body transform into one that you'd always envied from other healthier women.

We have put together quite a bit of information on what you need to know and do to become stronger and fitter than ever before. Once you get used to following the healthy steps we tell you to, it will just become a way of life for you. And this is definitely the kind of life you will be happier in.

Thanks again for purchasing this book, I hope you enjoy it!

information is without contract or any type of guarantee assurance.

The trademarks that are used are without any consent, and the publication of the trademark is without permission or backing by the trademark owner. All trademarks and brands within this book are for clarifying purposes only and are the owned by the owners themselves, not affiliated with this document.

Chapter 1:
How To Get Started Towards
A Healthy Body

The first step to getting healthy and building a stronger, fitter body is having the will to do so. Once you are determined on attaining that goal, you can definitely do it. And we are here to help you with this.

One thing women need to realize is that building their body is not the same as how men build theirs. The constitution of a male and female body is very different and they can never be built the same way. The only way that a woman can become as bulky as a male bodybuilder is if they use steroids. And that is not what we are looking for.

Women can build their bodies to become fitter and have well defined muscles but those muscles are still female muscles. So you need never worry about losing your feminine form while working those muscles. So keep such fears aside and get started.

First set your goals and make them attainable not impractical. This will help you in long term progress and you will know what you really want. As you work towards it, keep track of what you are doing so that you know where you stand. Keep a log of it and you will even notice where you might be going wrong.

Find out what state your body is in presently and take help from a professional to see what is suitable for you. Explore different options to find something that will work best for you. Know what your limits are and train in a way that doesn't over-work your body.

Once you decide what type of workout or training you are going to do, make changes according to the rest of your lifestyle as well. The first step is to make changes in your diet. Educate yourself about what you should be eating and what you should avoid. Don't follow any myths which will steer you in the wrong direction.

For instance, all fats are not bad for you. Fats are an important part of your diet as well as long as they are the good kind. Once you get the right kind of nutrition into your body, it will work optimally and help you reach the state you want.

Your body needs a minimum amount of calories each day which differs for people. One way to calculate your required intake is to multiply the weight of your body measured in pounds into 10. Then add 300 more calories to it if your lifestyle is not active, 500 calories if you are active on an average level and 800 if you live a very active life.

The number can vary a little around this depending on your metabolism as well. Just make sure that you take these calories from good sources like fruits, lean meat, etc.

The first three months of when you get started are crucial. This time helps you set a particular routine and you should track your progress as well.

Commit three to four days of the week to your training. Alternate days like Monday, Wednesday and then Friday, work well. You need to find exercises which burn fat and build muscle instead. Put in at least an hour on these days to see results.

The first month will be more about you getting acclimatized to all this. After that make sure to be rigorous and focused.

Always warm up before doing the hard stuff or you will injure yourself. Especially for those women who are really unfit and do not normally perform any physical exercise; it can be quite straining for the body. So make sure to loosen up your body and not cause any harm instead of improving it.

Stretching before a proper workout is very important. First get warmed up with a little aerobics like form of movement. Then do some dynamic stretching which could vary from hip rotations to butt kicks. Do the static stretches after you have finished working out and not before.

Your initial stretching should just be a start up and you should have enough energy to spend on your actual workout. Warm ups will prepare your body both mentally and physically for the workout.

There are three important aspects of to body building in women. The first is diet and nutrition. The second is cardiovascular exercises and the third is strength training. Incorporating these three in a proper manner into your lifestyle will make all the difference.

Cardio is one of the essential parts of your training. You can choose from a variety of forms like swimming, running, biking etc. Then really get into it so that it actually works on your body. One of the best methods that have gained popularity lately is interval training. For example run at a normal speed for about 15 minutes and then pick up the pace for 5 minutes and get back to a slow run again. Do this for about 3 cycles to make it effective. We will explain more about this later on.

The strength training part of your routine is what will build all that lean muscle for a leaner body. And building muscle will automatically burn fat as well. There are different exercises to make strength training very effective on your body.

Last but not the least, diet and nutrition will make a whole lot of difference. Find out what you have been doing wrong and start eating the right kinds of food in the right proportions. Creating a proper meal plan for you will go a long way. Consult an expert to help you get started.

Chapter 2:
Eating Healthy

Eating healthy food as a part of a balanced diet plan is one of the cornerstones of your journey towards good health. It is as important as the exercise that you need to do to get your body in shape. It's not about going on an intense starvation diet but about being disciplined and conscious of what you eat.

If you put in the wrong types of food in your body, the results will definitely not be the right ones. You need to know what exactly you are eating and how it will affect your body.

Try to eat home-cooked and healthy food as much as possible. When you do buy things from the stores, pay close attention to what they contain.

While most people think a good diet is about losing weight, you need to know that it isn't just about that. When you are trying to build a healthier body, it is also about gaining weight. The point is to lose the unwanted fats and gain healthy muscle weight. This can be done by eating the right type of food and keeping count of your calories.

Read on to know about different foods that will benefit you and those you should steer clear of. We will also tell you how to implement healthy eating habits in your daily life. It is very important to change your unhealthy eating habits. Just by doing this and even without the exercise, you will see a change in how your body feels.

You need the three macro-nutrients in your body no matter what anyone else says. Proteins, carbohydrates and fats are all necessary for different roles in your body.

Proteins are essential for building all that lean muscle you need to improve your body. The amino acids in proteins are required for a variety of different purposes by the body. The proteins will also repair the muscles which get damaged during your workouts and will help you get stronger. Some protein needs to be included in every meal.

Fats are another important part of your diet. Especially women seem to shy away from these like the plague. However this fear is misguided and needs to be corrected. The only fats that you need to avoid are all the Trans fat that is found in most packaged food.

Good fat gives you essential fatty acids which instead keep you feeling full for a longer time and help your body to function optimally by other means. What you need to avoid is eating too much fat. The fat gets stored in your body when there is just too much for the body to use and so it gets stored.

Carbohydrates are another misunderstood part of your diet. You just need to limit your intake of them. Complex carbs will leave you felling full for a longer time as they take longer to digest and they also contain many other nutrients which your body needs. The amount of carbohydrates your body needs will differ for different people.

Tips to eat healthy:

Get rid of any unhealthy food that you have lying around your house. Processed food, fried snacks, sodas, etc are all harmful to your body and have absolutely no benefits. Instead such foods are quite harmful and affect you in a negative way. Such junk food also cause mood and energy swings which have a negative impact on you.

Stock up your pantry with the right kind of food. Lots of fresh fruits and vegetables with good meat and fish is a must.

Make meal plans for your entire week to keep on track with what you will be eating.

Eat a healthy breakfast that will keep you going strong throughout the day. People who tend to skip breakfast also tend to gain more weight. A nutritious breakfast will get your metabolism going.

Eat regularly throughout the day to prevent unhealthy cravings and binge eating. A heavy breakfast, proper lunch and light dinner are the way to go. In between these you can have a small healthy snack every 2-3 hours to stay on track.

Eat the good type of carbohydrates and fats instead of the unhealthy ones. You may think that these words are synonymous with being unhealthy but they aren't. Eat complex carbohydrates like whole grains and beans instead of simple carbohydrates like white rice and sugary items.

The complex foods will keep you full with a lot of energy unlike the simple ones. Good fats are those found in plant oils like olive oil, omega-3 and 6 fatty acids from fish, soybean, etc. These contribute to your health unlike unhealthy fats from foods like butter, cookies and red meat.

Eat foods which improve bone health. Such foods will contain calcium, magnesium or vitamin D. Oatmeal, eggs, broccoli, sesame and beans are some such examples.

Add a proper amount of fiber to your diet. It is good for digestion, proper bowel movement, reduces the risk of heart diseases, etc. Fiber also helps you feel full for a longer time and you don't feel as hungry.

At least 25-30 grams of fiber should be consumed daily. You can eat more fibrous foods for breakfast and snacks in the form of food like oatmeal, carrots, whole grain bread, fruits, etc.

Keep control over your proportions. Don't overeat something just because it is said to be healthy. Too much of anything will always be unhealthy. Make sure to include all the necessary nutrients in your daily diet in a balanced way. You can't keep counting calories for the rest of your life. So instead keep note of your portions. Don't just pile your plates with food at every chance you get.

Try to eat as much organic food as possible. This will prevent accumulation of harmful substances like pesticides and other farming chemicals in your body.

Some Food that will help you in your fitness goals:

Foods that help in burning fat

Walnuts

Ginger

Oatmeal

Avocado

Salmon

Soybean

Flaxseed

Grapefruit

Honey

Eggs

Broccoli

Green tea

Lentils

Foods that help to build lean muscle

Beetroot

Brown rice

Oranges

Eggs

Milk

Quinoa

Spinach

Apples

Yoghurt

Olive oil

Sweet potatoes

Almonds

The above mentioned foods are just some of the important things that you should include in your diet. There are a lot of other healthy whole grains, fruits and vegetables that you can enjoy while you get into shape. Just make a good diet plan with these nutritious types of food and stay away from harmful junk food.

Chapter 3:
Cardiovascular Exercise

Cardiovascular exercises are equally important or even more than the strength training. Strength training is about getting fitter with better muscle definition. Cardio will kick things up for you and burn a whole lot of that excess fat. In fact do the strength workout first and then the cardio for it to be more effective.

The best way to go about cardio is high intensity interval training or HIIT, like we mentioned before. This has been found to be much more effective than the slow and steady pace most people go at.

This type of training involves alternative short periods of high intensity bouts of your exercise and then the normal pace again. This helps to use up more fat as energy in less time.

You get ample time to recover and then have enough energy to do the intense exercise for a few minutes. You might think that it won't work as well as a continuous period of intensely working out but you will be surprised. You'll be so worn out that you will realize just how effective HIIT is.

There are many ways to do your cardio other than normal exercises.

> Running is definitely the best option according to most people. You feel much better after a good run as it stimulates so all your happy hormones. Your heart rate kicks up, fats are burned and stamina really improves.

> Swimming is another versatile form of working out. Your entire body is worked on and you can actually have fun

while doing this particular activity. It's a great way to beat the heat in summer while you are burning the fats inside.

Bicycling is a great option that you can do on an indoor machine or enjoy outside. You can have fun while you workout with this form of cardio.

Aerobics is another great option that literally lets you dance your fats away. Start with a low intensity aerobic workout and move up as you get better. It tones your overall body and you really get your heart rate going.

Another stress relieving form is kick boxing. It improves your coordination and increases your body's flexibility as well. It burns a lot of calories with structured movements.

Skipping or jumping rope is another effective option that many women prefer. You can really workout with this one and make it fun too.

Good old walking is something anyone can do at any age. It works on your entire body and you can set your own pace. You can even do interval training with some walking and jogging alternatively.

Brisk walking is the most effective as opposed to a casual walk but either way it is a healthy form of exercise.

Chapter 4:
Strength Training

Strength training is extremely important for those women who don't just want to lose weight but want to build up their body with muscle. It does not mean that your body will turn into a bulky form like male body builders we normally see. There are different workouts to make sure you build muscle but retain that feminine aspect as well.

It uses resistance to increase muscle contraction and thus improve strength and endurance of the muscles. Strength training is a part of nearly any sport training, be it football or hockey. It helps to increase the level of performance of the athlete.

People who do weight bearing exercises are also known to be less prone to osteoporosis and their bones are much stronger than other.

Not only will you build muscle, you will automatically be burning fat as well. It boosts your metabolic rate which in turn boosts the rate that your body burns calories. It can help in making all your muscles, tendons and ligaments more strong and tough while bone density also increases.

The most effective exercises are compound, that is, they work on multiple muscles and joints. Some of these are squats and bench press. These exercises are extremely effective as they engage multiple parts. Do a couple sets of about 10 repetitions of each exercise. It is also important that you don't rest for too long in between each set or it won't be as effective.

When you are starting out with your strength training, there are a few things to keep in mind. Firstly learn the proper form of any exercise you are about to perform. This will give you the best results and avoid any mishaps.

Also don't start out beyond your capacity. Start with a few exercises that your body can actually tolerate and then move higher up on the levels. As you progress you can start adding more weights and make your training more challenging.

Different exercises concentrate on different parts of the body. Some compound exercises work on many parts together. Some good exercises for the shoulders are arm dumbbell press and handstand push ups. Rollouts and crunches really work well on your abs. Concentrate on exercises which deal with your problem areas in the beginning.

Some of the best strength exercises for beginners are squats, deadlifts, vertical and horizontal pushes, etc. Deadlifts are great for your back. Chin ups and bicep curls are good for the biceps. Triceps get worked up by push downs and dips.

You can work on your abs with crunches, leg raises, sit ups, etc. The front of your thighs will benefit from squats, lunges and leg presses. You can work on the back of the thighs with leg curls and squats.

Push ups, bench presses, chest fly's are good for the pectorals. Wrist curls work on your forearms. Your shoulders will benefit from front raises, military presses, shoulder presses, etc. Calve raises are effective to tone the calves.

When you do the compound exercises do 5 sets of 5 reps for effective movement. For muscle shaping movements do 8-12 reps each.

For the first 3-4 weeks your work outs will be relatively low intensity and with lighter loads.

Don't push yourself too much just as you start out. You can add more as you progress further. Then after these initial weeks you can go to a more advanced version of your workout from the initial primary form.

As you advance, your goal should be to increase the weights and intensity of your training. Things can only get better if you are just be persistent and determined.

Don't shy away from proper strength training thinking you will lose your attractiveness as a female. Instead your body will develop a more firm and toned look that makes it all the more better. Your metabolic rate increases and helps you maintain this better physical form as well.

Yoga is also another type of strength training and is very popular amongst women. This form of exercise has existed for centuries and has gained immense popularity over the past few years. It is a much more holistic approach to exercising and is very effective.

Not only does your body improve physically but also mentally. There are so many different aspects of yoga. If practised properly, yoga is known to have so many benefits. It helps the body to work at its optimum potential and gives immense peace of mind.

Other forms of strength training are Pilates, gymnastics, circuit training, etc. These can be done with the help with different equipment that have been developed over the years and also with nothing at all.

Chapter 5:
Guide To Execute Some Exercises
In A Correct Manner

While exercising is important, it is equally important to do it right. If you do them wrong they won't work as well and you might even seriously injure yourself.

It is very important to breathe properly while you workout. Inhale deeply and exhale through the mouth during exercising.

You should also make sure that you perform the exercises at a comfortable level. You need stress your body but not to a level that it is harmed instead of improved. Once you get the hang of regularly working out, you will see an improvement in your stamina and thus be able to do them at a better pace.

Squat jumps

Keep your feet about hip-width apart. Then bend the knees and get into squat position. Then press into your heels and jump up as you straighten your legs. Land back softly and continue the same way.

Walking push up

Keep your legs straight as you bend down and put your hands on the floor. Then walk out with your hands while keep your feet in the same place till your back is straight. Then do the push-up and pull your feet towards your hands this time and stand up again. Repeat this for a set.

Squats

Stand shoulder width apart and bend through your hips and knees till the hips reach knee level. Keep your upper back tight. Move your knees to the side and push your hips down. While going up push your hips up while keeping your back tight and knees out. Take a deep breath and repeat.

Hammer curls

Hold your weights while keeping your arms in a straight position by your sides. Then use your forearm to bring the weight up as your biceps contract. Keep your wrist in line with your arm. Once your hand comes in contact with your upper arm, wait for a second, squeeze and lower down again. Repeat.

Crunches

Lie down on a hard surface with your face up towards the ceiling. Bend your legs and put your hands behind your head. Then contract your abdominal muscles as you push up using your shoulders. Keep your neck straight and don't push up while straining your neck. Hold the position as you rise up for a second or two and then push down again. Repeat. Pull yourself up with your upper body and don't pull your head up with your hands. You will soon feel the burn in your abdominal region.

Lunges

Stand straight at first. Then take a big step forward with one leg and bend that knee to nearly ninety degrees. The leg at the back should put pressure on the toes as it bends down towards the floor. Then move back up and repeat. This works on most of the major muscles. Repeat a set on one leg and then another set on the opposite leg.

Push up

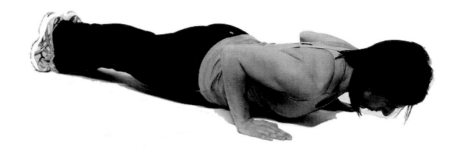

(Picture courtesy of Rance Costa – Flickr - https://www.flickr.com/photos/djrome/4253058200/)

Stay face down on the floor on the support of your hands and feet. Keep your hands a little more than shoulder width apart and your back straight. Now slowly bend your arms and lower your chest till it nearly touches the floor. Wait for a second and straighten your arms to move up again. Then repeat for a set. When you start out with push ups, you can begin by starting on a chair and then get down on the floor once you get the hang of it.

These are just some exercises. There are many others that you can implement in your workouts. For example:

Dumbbell military press

Barbell rows

Barbell curls

Hanging leg raise

Seated leg extensions

Seated leg curls

Cable crossovers

Leg press

Leg extensions

Dumbbell shoulder press

Lat pull downs

Ab roller

Deadlifts with dumbells or kettle bells

Barbell bench press

Dumbell bench press

Dumbell Flyes (below)

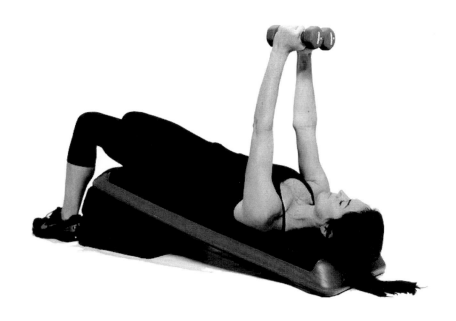

(Picture courtesy of Rance Costa – Flickr - https://www.flickr.com/photos/djrome/4253061232/)

There's just so many that you can do. Just make sure to do the exercises in the right form and it is best to get the help of a trainer when starting out. They will help you through the whole process and if not for the long run, take a few sessions just to get proper guidance.

Chapter 6:
Common Mistakes

Here are some of the most common workout mistakes that you should avoid;

Just cardio is not going to work. Resistance training is a very important part of your work out and is essential for building muscle. The more muscle you build, the more fats will be burnt.

Don't do the same workout every day and don't work out every day either. Keep a little variety and work out on alternate days. This gives your muscles time to relax and repair.

Don't miss out on the necessary water intake. It is extremely important and will flush out all those toxins from your body. If you get dehydrated you won't be able to get through your entire workout and end up fainting.

Keep your form right during every workout. The wrong form will give you none or wrong results.

Don't avoid food after working out. Your body needs some proteins after it has worked so hard.

Also, don't eat a low calorie diet. Like we have said before, calories are important. You should just stick to a limit and count the calories you consume. They should be the right kind from the right type of food and not from junk food which will harm your body.

Don't set unrealistic expectations from yourself and your body. Each person is unique and will have

different results from different workouts. Some people might see faster results than you do and their bodies might appear better to you. But what's important is to be consistent and do the best that you can.

Don't follow random fad diets. Eat the right kinds of food in a well proportioned way. Consult a good dietician for proper guidance. When you need to build muscle you need a lot of different foods. Most fads are nonsensical and absolutely bad for your body. Be healthy and fit not skinny.

Do not skip breakfast. We just can't emphasise enough on how important this one meal is. It has been proved time and again that women who eat a healthy breakfast will, any day, be fitter than ones who skip this meal. You will actually burn more fats during the day by eating this meal properly. Skipping breakfast will only cause you to over eat later in the day.

Don't exercise for spot reduction. It really isn't possible to just lose fat in one part of the body by doing exercises that only concentrate on them. It is important to do a workout which works on the overall body to deal with any of your problem areas as well.

Don't avoid weights. There are just too many women who shy away from weights and it does not make any sense. Weights will not give women that bulky male body they seem to fear they will get. Women are built in a different way and just can't get that way. Weights will increase your muscle mass but you will get toned not bulked up.

Don't just eat any so called fat free and low sugar foods in excessive quantities.

Sometimes even older women suddenly have the urge to take up bodybuilding. If they are in good health and their body can sustain it then there is no reason not to. The older generation should get a proper medical consult before embarking on any training. A full assessment of their health is a good idea to make sure they are up for the workout they take up. The intensity and frequency of their workout should be in proportion to their health assessment result.

Get proper supervision especially for strength training. Engaging in it without any guidance can cause serious injuries which will be much harder to deal with. Proper guidance will prevent any torn ligaments and twisted ankles. You can benefit from the guidance of these trained professionals to get the most of your work out and get the best results instead of harming your body

Conclusion

Thank you again for purchasing this book!

Now that you have read through all the information in this book, you should know quite a lot about what you need to do to get a healthy body.

I have put everything in a simple and concise manner that should help you to get fit in no time at all. Follow the different tips and start exercising regularly to get amazing results in no time at all.

Working to get a healthy body will help you live a healthy life with a much happier mental state as well. You can be more confident and things just get better from there. Your body will be in its optimal health zone and you can lead a good, long life.

Finally, if you enjoyed this book, then I'd like to ask you for a favor, would you be kind enough to leave a review for this book on Amazon? It'd be greatly appreciated!

Want more books?

Would you love books delivered straight to your inbox every week?

Free?

How about non-fiction books on all kinds of subjects?

We send out e-books to our loyal subscribers every week to download and enjoy!

All you have to do is join! It's so easy!

Just visit the link below to sign up and then wait for your books to arrive!

www.LibraryBugs.com

Enjoy :)

Thank you and good luck!

Made in United States
North Haven, CT
16 October 2023

42812318R00019

A Step-By-Step Bodybuilding For Women Training Guide For Beginners On Building The Strongest, Fittest Female Body Ever

You're about to discover how to start out, bodybuilding for women and what a great sport/pastime it is to take up. Health and fitness is one of the most important things in our lives and if we aren't healthy then we risk getting diseases and living less fulfilling lives.

In "Bodybuilding For Women" I take you through the basics of starting out bodybuilding, from the first day you step into a gym, to getting the right foods in your kitchen. Everyone knows how important it is to be healthy and fit in order to live a good life. But there are too many people who do nothing to get this.

But I can only tell you what to do, all you have to do then is do it! A healthy body will help you live a healthier and happier life. You can only get that kind of body if you are willing to work for it. And although it may seem hard to follow the steps, the result is definitely worth it...

ISBN 9781534812741

90000 >

9 781534 812741